The Pria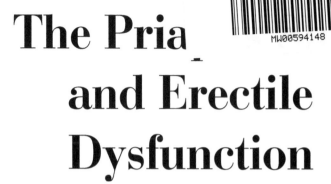 and Erectile Dysfunction

What You Need to Know About the P-Shot

The Priapus Shot and Erectile Dysfunction

What You Need to Know About the P-Shot

By Phyllis C. Okereke, MD

ISBN: 978-1-945446-05-4

YouSpeakIt
PUBLISHING
The Easy Way
to Get Your Book
Done Right

www.YouSpeakItPublishing.com

Acknowledgments

I am grateful to Charles Runnel, MD, who developed the Priapus Shot, also called the *P-Shot*®, and trained most of the doctors who offer this procedure. He continues to mentor me and provided the springboard for this book.

Thanks to my colleagues at BodyLogicMD, who collectively offer an easily available source of knowledge and experience. Thank you to Patrick Savage, the architect of BodyLogicMD, an organization that makes the delivery of healthcare both effective and fun for practitioners and their clients.

I would like to thank Dr. Charles Webb and Matt Lowman for their great ability to draw out the best in people and motivate them to get started.

Thank you to my publisher, YouSpeakIt, for making this book a reality.

I would like to thank Chioma Okereke, my daughter, whose idea it was to write this book and whose constant encouragement throughout the process made this endeavor possible.

I would also like to thank my husband, John Okereke, my best friend, sounding board, and most ardent supporter.

Contents

Introduction

This book on the Priapus treatment, or the P-Shot, was written to provide basic information to men who are suffering from erectile dysfunction (ED). It is especially helpful for men who recognize the impact of their dysfunction on themselves and on their spouses, coworkers, and friends. This book is meant to guide the reader to understand that he is not alone: ED is a common problem that can be caused by a number of contributing health issues.

The author also intends to inform the reader about the options that are available to help him with this problem. The first chapter explains that ED is not an issue that is limited to the erectile tissue. It can be an indication of a more serious problem occurring elsewhere in the body, which can be properly addressed once it is identified.

In addition, this book will describe the Priapus Shot and answer many, if not all, of the questions that a man may have about receiving treatment for ED, especially regarding the P-Shot. Many of the sections in this book are based on the questions we are asked by potential patients who come into the author's clinic, BodyLogicMD of Houston, for a consultation. The information is given in a straightforward and accessible manner, to be of assistance to men everywhere who may have the same questions.

Providers' staff can also benefit from this book by educating themselves about the Priapus Shot, which will put them in a better position to answer patients' questions. At BodyLogicMD of Houston, we have had many men come in because they can't get the answers to their questions elsewhere. Having the answers can give a patient the confidence he needs to try the Priapus Shot.

This guide can also be given to spouses and significant others, especially if they notice problems that their partners are not willing to discuss. By reading this book, a partner may be more capable of engaging in conversation with a man and encouraging him to seek help.

This book informs readers about some of the major causes of ED, the associated conditions, the contributing habits or lifestyle factors that could contribute or worsen ED, and what can be done to remedy it.

The P-Shot is thoroughly discussed: not only is it one of the least invasive ways to treat ED, it's also less fraught with complications if done properly. I strongly recommend this treatment for ED because it is minimally invasive, unlike ED pills. For example, a patient won't become alarmed and call his doctor in the middle of the night because his vision starts going. A patient doesn't need to be concerned about using the P-Shot treatment if he is on nitroglycerin. There are no medical contraindications beyond the typical concerns raised by any kind of injection.

Overall, this book seeks to provide the reader with the basic material he or she needs to know about what is going on in ED and how the P-Shot can be used to improve erectile function.

The best way to read this guide is to begin at the beginning.

CHAPTER ONE

It's More Common
Than You Think

FACING THE FACTS

Many people are faced with a health issue and yet are not ready to deal with it, don't know what to do about it, or don't understand that they can get help for it. It can be very frustrating to have a health issue that doesn't easily and immediately respond to treatment. It can be even more difficult to live with a health concern and not know that there are options to be considered.

When a man doesn't know he can get help, he can suffer with a problem for months or even for years. The knowledge that this is a common problem and that it can be taken care of, if the right information is available, makes this condition much easier to tolerate.

The problem of erectile dysfunction (ED) is extremely common and, fortunately, the treatment for it is available. Most sufferers don't know that a treatment is accessible or that they can deal with the issue at all.

The Psychological Effects of ED

The psychological effects of ED are not limited to only the individual who has the problem.

- When you are unable to perform during sexual intercourse, it can affect your confidence.

- Your doubts and dissatisfaction can be projected onto people around you, especially your spouse or significant other, and you may withdraw from interaction with this individual.

- ED can lead to irritable behavior or increasing anxiety and depression.

- Your reactions might expand beyond intimate relationships to affect other people, such as coworkers, friends, and even acquaintances.

Fear and worry can affect many aspects of your life when your body won't perform the way you want it to.

Embarrassment

You may be embarrassed about having this intimate problem. However, this condition is very common and a number of men, starting from a very young age, experience ED. It might be caused by a psychological problem; ED can both result from and compound underlying psychological problems. If you have been under a lot of stress, whether it's from physical overwork or mental illness or traumatic life experiences, you can have this problem.

At the other extreme, a medical practitioner may have older patients whose tissues are beginning to age, either faster than they might have because of lifestyle choices, or because of the passing years. A lot of men are simply experiencing the effects of aging. However, help can be found for these issues as well. If you are willing to face the facts and understand the possibilities of overcoming ED, you can then go on to address the causes head on. Eventually, most patients do find a resolution to their problem. ED is not a life sentence, and it shouldn't be seen as such.

Treatment Options for ED

There are many treatment options available for patients with ED. These include pharmaceutical medications, and you can find blue pills like Viagra and other cures that can be seen on television.

Sometimes the treatment can involve counseling the patient. The man may need to face the fact that whatever issue is causing his ED, it can help to address, rather than avoid, the problem. For some men, a lot more than one consultation is needed.

For example, the cause of ED may be a hormonal deficiency that should be addressed. Lifestyle choices can affect hormonal balance, so the lifestyle issues that could impact the production of hormones should also be considered.

Some people will need more extensive procedures, which may involve injecting drugs or taking herbal products to get an erection.

And finally, there is the procedure known as a P-Shot, which is an injection of platelet-rich plasma. This treatment works completely differently because it helps enable the man's tissues to perform better.

Reluctance to Attempt New Treatments

For most men, past failures to overcome ED can arise from either having used drug treatments that didn't work for them, or from having implants that didn't work. These failures can make them unwilling to try anything else, even when they are just a step away from getting the correct treatment for their problem.

The important thing to begin to solve any problem is for a person to understand that they do, in fact, have a problem. Once they understand that there is a problem, they should try to find out what is available to deal with it. Identifying a problem and thinking it's the end of the world does not help because it just leads to more depression and anxiety. Identifying a problem and trying to find out what is available to deal with this problem is strongly recommended because almost every problem has an answer. You simply need to find the right answer.

The same applies to ED. There are plenty of opportunities for treatment of this condition. Accept that there is a problem, and look for help.

ROOT CAUSES OF ERECTILE DYSFUNCTION

When we address the health issues that can lead to ED, we can limit the ED that arises from these causes. For example, if a man has a lifestyle that reduces his risk of developing diabetes, at the same time he will be reducing the risk of ED, which is a secondary effect of diabetes. High blood pressure is exactly the same kind of underlying cause that can be helped by making healthful choices.

Most chronic diseases stem from our lifestyle choices. Taking care about what you eat, whether you smoke or drink alcohol, or what type of exercise you do will limit the chances of developing diabetes, high blood pressure, or autoimmune diseases.

Diabetes

Diabetes is a disease that affects your entire body. Every tissue in your body that has a blood supply can have a complication caused by diabetes. One of the tissues that is most commonly affected by diabetes is the small blood vessels. Erectile tissue is supplied by small blood vessels. If the small blood vessels are damaged by diabetes, there will not be sufficient blood flow to the penile area, and the result will be ED.

Unfortunately, what is happening to the erectile tissue is also happening to every other organ in the body. When someone has ED from diabetes, they should also assume that they have a similar issue in every other tissue in their body, including the heart and the brain. ED is a sign that things are not going well inside the body. In this case, we should not be thinking only about ED, but also about the heart, the brain, the kidneys, and every other organ in our body.

In that case, every effort should be made to control the diabetes. Diabetes can usually be controlled by changing lifestyle habits, especially diet and nutrition.

What do you eat?

It is not healthy to have a fast food diet every day. It is also unhealthy to have a diet that is filled with simple starches. When I say simple starches, I mean refined carbohydrates, such as:

- Table sugar, corn syrup, molasses
- Refined grains such as white flour
- Fruit juices

These types of foods should be limited or completely eliminated, if possible. They can be replaced with foods that you can learn to enjoy:

- Vegetables
- Fruits
- Protein

Apart from eating healthful foods, we should also exercise, because exercise helps our bodies use calories. By exercising and improving blood flow throughout our bodies, we also increase our ability to use sugar. Ingesting excess sugar is what causes the pancreas to make more insulin, and excess insulin is toxic to the body. Sometimes by giving diabetics insulin, we may not be doing them any favors. Even though we are controlling the level of blood sugar, we are also introducing something that has a negative effect on the body and is probably unnecessary.

High Blood Pressure

High blood pressure usually begins in the small blood vessels of the body. The cells lining the smallest blood vessels in the body are the cells that make the substances that allow our blood vessels to dilate. When the blood vessels are elastic and able to dilate, blood pressure stays normal. The high pressure eventually affects the muscle walls of the blood vessels, which means they can't relax when they are supposed to relax. When the blood vessels are unable to expand, then blood pressure rises, and this will cause more damage to the small blood vessels in tissues, including the erectile tissues. This compounds the problem.

The small blood vessels may be affected by inflammation, which can be caused by lifestyle choices. There is a saying that the commonest form of suicide is with a fork and knife, because of the powerful effects of diet upon our well-being. Many health problems are related to what we eat.

If a man with high blood pressure also has ED, this is a warning that the small blood vessels in the heart, the brain, and the kidneys are also in trouble. ED is more than a psychological or sexual performance issues: it is like a canary in a coal mine. It shows that something is happening in the tissues inside the body.

Luckily for us, there is an external manifestation, which if dealt with, can lead to improvement. That's why I stress to my patients that it doesn't matter which procedure they choose, it is the lifestyle changes that can correct the diseases of the blood vessels in the rest of their body and maintain the positive results of treatment.

Autoimmune Diseases

Again, I want to stress the fact that ED is the end result of an unhealthy damaging process that has been going on in the body for a period of time. Autoimmune diseases affect blood vessels and cause the inflammation that increases the amount of free radicals in the body, which destroy tissues. Autoimmune diseases will destroy tissues in different parts of the body, including erectile tissues. They also are preventable by lifestyle changes. Even if someone comes from a family with a strong history of this disease, all they truly have is the *potential* to develop that disease. For that disease to manifest in the individual, they have to do something to turn on the gene. What we do to turn on such bad genes depends on our lifestyle choices.

If we eat a lot of refined carbohydrates or processed foods with additives, this diet can stimulate our immune system in the wrong way. Some of those foods can cause allergies, such as wheat, if a person has a gluten sensitivity, but it also goes beyond that. When the intestines are stressed, particles of food that shouldn't get through are able to pass through the walls of the intestine, in a condition called "leaky gut."

The cells of the walls of the intestine are supposed to be arranged in a very tight formation; they have what we call tight junctions. When we eat things we shouldn't eat, those tight junctions are weakened. Particles of food get through the walls, and the body reacts to those particles. Some of those particles attach to the proteins in our body, and our immune cells try to get rid of them.

Any tissue in the body can be affected. If the gland that makes insulin, the pancreas, is affected then diabetes can develop. If the joints are affected then you can get arthritis. And autoimmune diseases can also affect the blood vessels. To be able to deal with ED, you have to control what is causing the autoimmune disease in the first place. Otherwise, it is like blowing away the smoke instead of putting out the fire.

Injury to the Area — Surgical or Accidental

Injury to the penile area can occur in a number of ways:

- Surgery and radiation treatment for prostate conditions

- Cycling, particularly on a racing bike with a narrow saddle

- Contact sports, and neglecting to wear protective gear, can present problems

- Accident that affects the penile area

- Vasectomy and hormonal imbalance as an unintended result

- Drug use, either prescribed or for recreational use

ED may occur as a result of prostate surgery for prostate cancer or an enlarged prostate. This may be an unavoidable problem because the patient has a serious condition that requires treatment. In a case like this, we need to revive the tissue to the highest degree we can with everything available to us.

Certain sports like cycling can damage the penile artery or nerve that supplies blood to the erectile tissue. The narrow seat of a racing bike, or contact with the top tube that connects the front of the bike to the seat, can cause numbness in the penis. Male cyclists can choose seats that are more padded or even wear padded bicycle pants. If you are a cyclist and you are going to be riding for a long time, you need to use gear that will limit the chance of injury.

For other types of contact sports, it's good for a man to wear proper protective gear. If a baseball player, for example, is hit in the groin by a fastball, he can sustain injury that is quite extensive.

In any instance of penis injury, we need to treat and heal the tissue around the area in order to minimize the effect of the trauma.

Another problem is that some men who have had vasectomies might have suffered damage to the nerve or blood supply to the area as a possible complication. Limiting the blood supply to the testes can affect hormone production, which is needed for erectile function. When someone has a vasectomy, they should be forewarned that this is an issue that could arise. They do need proper follow-up with their physician to make sure the hormones are at the right level. They don't need to wait until they develop ED before they start addressing these issues. Sometimes, just correcting the hormonal imbalance will correct the ED fully or significantly.

If a man has ED and suffers from hormonal imbalance, even if he is using ED medication he will not experience the full benefit of the drug. This is because the blue pill interacts with naturally occurring hormones in the body to be effective, and if the hormones are not present, the drug will not work.

Medications prescribed to treat other diseases can also have negative effects on erectile function:

- Certain blood pressure medications
- Antidepressants
- Pain medications
- Antianxiety drugs
- Antiepileptics
- Antihistamines
- Nonsteroidal anti-inflammatory drugs (NSAIDs)

- Parkinson's disease medication
- Stomach or prostate cancer drugs
- Cancer treatment drugs
- Street drugs, such as amphetamines, cocaine, and marijuana

PSYCHOLOGICAL CAUSES AND EFFECTS

The way we differentiate ED caused by psychological issues from ED based on a physical problem in the erectile tissue is by asking if a man experiences morning erections. If he does, then his inability to have an erection in an intimate sexual encounter is psychological. A man who suffers from a physical problem in the erectile tissue will not have morning erections.

Psychological issues can lead to ED:

- Depression and anxiety
- Past history of sexual abuse
- Anger management issues
- Relationship problems with an intimate partner

Depression and Anxiety

Depression can cause ED, as can many drugs used for the treatment of depression. Some of the drugs used for depression lower testosterone levels, and low testosterone is associated with ED. So depression should be addressed and treated and attention should be paid to the choice of drugs used in the treatment of these individuals.

For men who develop ED either from medical problems or from trauma or even surgery, it can be a devastating blow to their ego and their perception of themselves as whole. Many of them feel ashamed to even talk about it. Even when they go to a doctor, and even if a doctor asks directly, some will try to suppress the problem, which can increase their depression. Whenever they find themselves in a sexual situation, the anxiety over whether they will be able to perform increases their depression, and that makes the ED even worse.

The other problem may be that they will take this psychological baggage outside the privacy of their homes. They may react to situations they shouldn't react to, as though they feel the world is against them. They may walk around with a chip on their shoulders. Some of them become withdrawn, and their friends may wonder what's going on with this person.

At work, if a coworker says "Hi," or "Good morning," this person may respond by growling, "What's good about it?"

The coworker or the friend who doesn't understand what is going with this individual may feel slighted, and that can generate emotional discomfort for both the person with ED and their coworkers or friends.

For a family man, most of the time, it is their significant other and their children who take the brunt of his irritability. Family members are surprised by the changes in this previously loving man that they all knew, but who has suddenly become an angry, grumpy individual who is hard to live with. This not only makes the individual with ED suffer from the health issue, but also from the guilt of causing unhappiness in his family.

Depression and anxiety can lead to ED, and ED creates more depression and anxiety, in a vicious cycle that is difficult to break.

Past History of Sexual Abuse

Many people who were sexually, psychologically, or even physically abused as young men or even as children have regular psychological, depressive issues, and these can lead to sexual problems, including ED.

A past history of sexual abuse can be devastating to the psyche of the individual, causing problems not only for the abused individual but also for everyone around him. Some men will act out, while others will internalize the abuse, and these are the men who are more likely to have issues with depression, ED, heart disease, and other types of chronic illnesses.

When young males go for ED assessment, it is very important to rule out a history of possible abuse because that will affect the result that you will eventually achieve by treatment. If you give only a physical treatment, and this person has some deep mental issues, then you're not going to get the best results. But if these issues are addressed concurrently with whatever is being done to treat the ED directly, then the results can be much more impressive than when treating only a small portion of the problem.

The problem causing ED might be more complicated than what we can see on the surface. The individual could have forgotten a past event that could be a major contributing factor to what is going on now.

Anger Management Issues

Patients with ED may have anger management issues, which can affect both work and family life. The ED should therefore be treated to preserve professional and family life and overall psychological well-being of the individual.

More depression, anxiety, or anger makes the ED worse, and this causes more depression and anxiety.

One thing makes the other worse, and the problem is thus continuously propagated.

Include questions in the initial meeting with a client to gently learn about any psychological issues that may be underlying their problems with ED.

CHAPTER *TWO*

TWO

The Good News: You Can Do Something About It!

HOW TO ASK FOR HELP

Many people with problems do not know how to ask for help, so never seem to get the help that they need. Whatever problem you have, be it psychological or physiological, you need to get relevant information to manage that problem. To get that information, you have to be able to ask for help. It is important for people with or manage whatever problem they may have, be it physiological or psychological or some other kind of crisis. You have to be able to ask for help. It is important for people with any type of health issue to ask for help and be able to get it.

To ensure that the process goes smoothly, it's a good idea to be prepared:

- Online research can narrow down your choice of doctor or clinic to give you the help you need.

- Educate yourself about the possible options that may be offered

- Have a list of questions at every stage, to be sure you don't forget a relevant issue

- Prepare yourself for the consultation with past medical records and other relevant information

- Maintain a positive attitude toward getting help

- Bring a significant other or friend to the consultation to ensure no detail is missed

Online Research

One advantage we all have today is that there is a lot of information available to anyone on the Internet, from WebMD to Wikipedia to Doctor Google and to groups of people who have had the same issues. Some people do not mind sharing their experiences. A lot of physicians or practitioners who offer different procedures offer at least some summarized form of what they can do about different issues online.

Getting information about the issue and then making an informed decision on what to do, or at least asking for help from someone who could help you decide what to do, is important. You can find a lot of information if you spend the time and effort. Some online information can be confusing or straight-out deceptive or wacky, but you can also find some very good, relevant information that can help you take the first step to seek help.

At the same time, the problem with online research is that you don't want to believe everything you see or read. So you have to be able to have a good analytical mind. If you don't think you can sort through the information yourself, then ask a family member, a friend, or a healthcare practitioner who may be in a completely different field. Many professional have some education about these issues and can direct you to the right and safe way to go.

Learning What Options Your Doctor Can Offer

After you have done research and decided which doctor or practitioner you would like to see, the first thing to do is to call the doctor's office, or at least send an email and ask for someone at the office to reach out to you. You should be able to give a brief account of why you need to be seen.

You do not necessarily have to give a detailed medical history to the receptionist or medical assistant, but at least let them know, "I need to see the doctor about such-and-such procedure," or "to discuss certain issues."

However, if the person on the other end is trained enough to accept salient information from you, then give it. All medical offices must comply with HIPAA (Health Insurance Portability and Accountability Act of 1996), which means that everyone who works at the office has to follow procedures that ensure the safety and privacy of your health information.

It is important to be precise when describing your needs. So the more information you can give early on, the easier it will be for you to be scheduled appropriately. Usually, a medical office will want to know if you would like to come in for a consultation, because that is the only way a doctor or a healthcare professional or practitioner can obtain the information to know exactly what is going on and assign or recommend the correct and most effective treatment for you. In addition, if you have done your research, at your consultation you can ask salient and relevant questions of the provider and get relevant answers.

When you go to see a doctor, have your questions ready, because of the limited time you can spend with him or her. Even if it is an hour, one hour goes very quickly when you dealing with a serious concern. But if you have done your research and know what you want to know more about, the chances of covering all your questions are higher.

Should you decide to give more detailed information when you call the health provider's office, be truthful and sincere: tell them exactly what's going on. Don't waste their time and your time trying to wrap things up in vague terms that nobody understands. Most medical offices have dealt with a lot of different problems. Nothing is novel to them.

Getting Ready for the Consultation

To get ready for the consultation, apart from having your questions ready, there may be certain tests you have been given in the past, and the doctor may need to look at them to get the whole picture. If you are on medications, bring in a list; that is important information. Some offices will send you a health questionnaire before you come in for an appointment: take some time to complete the questionnaire. Be truthful with your answers, and give as much detail as you possibly can. Arrive for the consultation with an open mind and the belief that you're going to be able to get answers and advice that will help to resolve the situation.

Some people make an appointment to see a doctor or healthcare professional and yet still believe they are not going to get any help or see any improvement in their conditions. We know that thought has a strong effect on health outcomes. Being very positive about whatever is going on with you improves your chances of getting good results, because being positive releases positive hormones, and positive hormones improve the health of your body. Believe you're going to get something good out of your consultation, and then you will.

It is important to bring someone with you for the consultation. Some men, because they are embarrassed and stressed about their ED, miss a lot of what is being said to them, and others forget things that their spouse or their significant other may be able to help them to remember.

As stated earlier, with ED, the same process that can affect the small blood vessels of the erectile tissue can also affect the small blood vessels of the brain, the kidneys, and the heart. The patient's memory may not be as good as it used to be. Having someone with you at the appointment can help ensure that everyone knows what's going on and increases the chances of your getting the most out of it.

ADDRESSING THE ROOT CAUSES

Why Address the Root Cause?

If you do not address the root cause of a problem, you are probably just wasting your time and effort in treating only the surface symptoms. An example would be if a house were on fire. If, instead of putting out the fire, you spend your effort blowing away the smoke, as soon as you clear the smoke, more smoke would come from the fire. It is nothing more than an exercise in futility.

This also applies to our health. Before healthcare professionals can put a name to a disease — that is, diagnose and assign a code — they will need to look into the problems in the body that are flying under the radar, so to speak. If it's high blood pressure or diabetes, for instance, you will never get control of the ED or any other problems until you have dealt with those important underlying causes.

Dealing With Chronic Stress

We now know that chronic stress is one of the greatest health risks anyone can have. Chronic stress affects not only your emotional behavior, but also your whole body. It affects your hormones and how your cells use nutrients from foods or supplements. Stress affects the function of every cell in the body, and therefore every organ in your body. So if someone's ED is due to chronic stress, then the source of the chronic stress should be identified and dealt with.

There are different ways to deal with chronic stress. Some stresses can be avoided. Others cannot, but we can change the way we react to them. We can also support the body in ways that allow the body to survive the effects of chronic stress so that it does not take the whole person down. We know that chronic stress can cause many chronic diseases, from diabetes to high blood pressure to cancer, as well as autoimmune diseases. Therefore the chronic stress must be dealt with first, before the ED can be successfully addressed.

Avoiding Injuries

Accidental trauma may be preventable, such as by wearing appropriate protective gear when involved in contact sports, or even for sports like tennis or baseball where there is a possibility of a projectile hitting the groin area. Wear protective gear when you are involved in such activities.

Trauma to cyclists will usually come from extended compression to the blood or nerve circulation to the pelvic tissues. A good padded seat is important, as previously mentioned. You should spend time and money getting a proper seat that will limit the amount of injury that could occur in the area.

Recovering From Surgery

Unfortunately, for men who have had surgery for prostate cancer or an enlarged prostate, although the surgeon tries as much as possible to limit the damage to surrounding tissues, tissue damage can still occur. However, when it is a choice between saving a life and preserving erectile function, most people will choose life and then deal with ED later on. These patients do not have much control over ED caused by surgery.

Choosing Health Over Poor Lifestyle Choices

For ED due to chronic disease, chronic stress, or accidental trauma, the individual has a huge role to play in prevention and protecting themselves. As mentioned earlier, most chronic diseases are self-made and can be addressed by making changes in your lifestyle.

OTHER PROCEDURES COMPARED WITH THE P-SHOT

There are many options available for dealing with ED. The procedure you have and the procedure that will produce the best results will depend on the root cause of your ED. These procedures are readily available. Whether you are given pills or injections or P-Shots or implants, the decision regarding which one to apply in any individual case depends on what has caused the problem in the first place and what is available to you. Some treatments work better than others, and some will take more time to get results, while others will give only transient results. Some procedures are more invasive than others, and some will use the natural healing abilities of your body to rejuvenate the erectile tissue to deal with the ED.

Medications

Medications for ED will be more effective if you are also addressing any chronic disease that would have predisposed you to ED in the first place. For example, a diabetic can apply healthy lifestyle changes including healthy nutrition and exercise, which will improve blood sugar management.

There is a substance made in your body called *nitric oxide*. Nitric oxide causes the blood vessels in different parts of the body to dilate. This is what happens during an erection: blood vessels dilate. However, ED medicines may not work in a good number of people who are unable to produce this compound. The other disadvantage of ED medications is that they need to be taken every time a sexual encounter is about to occur. This could create additional stress if you are wondering whether you will get the results you need when you need them.

Under certain conditions these medications may not work at all. For example, if you have very low testosterone, ED medications may be ineffective. This is because testosterone is involved in the production of nitric oxide through interaction with another hormone: estrogen. So if you have low testosterone, you may not produce adequate amounts of nitric oxide. In such a case, the ED medicine may not be very helpful. Diabetes causes direct damage to blood vessels, but it also lowers testosterone production, further impacting ED. You would need to have an assessment to determine where your hormone levels are and work with a practitioner to address the hormonal deficiency simply and effectively.

Of course just taking testosterone will also not solve the problem. You need to have an assessment to see why you have low testosterone.

Is it due to old age, chronic disease like high blood pressure or diabetes, or is it because of chronic stress?

Is it because of toxins that come from processed foods?

By toxic foods I do not only mean foods that have had arsenic or insecticides spread on them; I mean foods that are toxic to the body just by their nature, for example, processed foods or foods with additives, artificial coloring, or trans-fats. These foods affect the way your body functions, such as production of your hormones. They have a very negative effect on the way your body works.

So just popping an ED pill may not give the results that you need because coexisting, predisposing health issues may not have been addressed. If you have been put on an ED pill or any other ED medication, you still need to address all the other health issues that will help the medication work more effectively.

Medications can also have systemic complications. For example, there may be certain types of medications you are taking that would have a negative reaction with Viagra. These could include serious side effects like a drop in blood pressure.

People have also experienced other complications:

- Low blood pressure
- Loss of vision
- Prolonged erection, priapism with the danger of more tissue damage if not released immediately
- Interaction with other drugs used for heart disease (e.g., nitroglycerine)

In this situation, you are taking a medication to help a local area that may have far-reaching complications for the rest of your body.

Injections

When injected locally, certain substances can cause *dilatation* or the expansion of the blood vessels in erectile tissues. The injected substance may be either Trimex or Bimix. Trimix and Bimix are a mixture of two or three drugs compounded by a compounding pharmacy for penile injection.

This, however, requires you to inject yourself every time you expect to have a sexual encounter. This is cumbersome and adds an additional layer of stress, and can lead to frustration with the whole process.

Injections don't really deal with the root cause of ED. They are a very temporary fix, a Band-Aid: they give relief, but do not deal with what is causing the ED in the first place.

Penile Pumps

You may also get some improvement in erection by using a penile pump. These devices create negative pressure and by doing so allow more blood to flow into the erectile tissue.

The effect of the pump is also transient because after a short while, the blood flows away from the erectile tissue, and the ED problem persists. You would need to repeat using the pump every time sexual intimacy is wanted. Some men do pumping in between sexual encounters, and some minimal longer-lasting effect could be obtained after extended use. However, in general, the penile pump used alone is not effective for any significant or long-lasting result. Our clinic advises using the pump in combination with the P-Shot to augment results.

Surgery

Surgery would be an option if you have had physical trauma, whether accidental or from complications of surgery, or in the case of some severe form of ED. Surgery is also used for penile enlargement. In this case, an implant, usually an artificial material, is placed into the penis to help keep it erect or increase its size. Like any surgery, the procedure can be complicated even in the best of hands. Problems can arise either during or any time after the surgery.

Whenever a foreign object is implanted into the body there is a very strong potential for infection, usually around the object. This could mean that the implant would need to be removed. When this happens, there is more scarring in the surrounding tissues, which can make the dysfunction much worse than it originally was. Surgery is an invasive procedure and also more expensive than other methods.

If you suffer from moderate ED, even if it is having a major psychological effect on you, surgery may not prove to be a good solution when the benefits are weighed against the chances of complications and all potential risks. Penile implants are not always advised, even you are willing to accept the risks that come with the procedure.

A number of my patients have had penile implants removed, and now they are trying to get treatment for their original ED condition, in addition to treatment for the complications of surgery, particularly scarring that was caused by the penile implants. Most surgeons will be unwilling to perform a procedure on a patient in which the risks outweigh the benefits.

None of the above procedures enhance your body's ability to heal itself. The penile implant, if there are no complications, could have a long-lasting effect; however, ED medications, penile injections, and the pump all have very transient effects. The patient still has to live with the fact that any time they need to have an erection, they will have to use something to achieve it. This has a psychological effect on a patient and affects his sex drive. I think anyone would prefer to think that, whenever they need to, they will be ready for a sexual encounter.

CHAPTER *THREE*

PRP and the
P-Shot Procedure

PLATELET-RICH PLASMA: DEFINED

Platelet-Rich Plasma (PRP) therapy is a procedure in which the healing power of the body — in particular, the stem cells present in the patient's own body — are harnessed to heal any part of the body. This is important because we each have the potential to heal ourselves when the conditions are right.

In these procedures, the PRP, which is the part of the blood without the red blood cells, is obtained from the patient and then injected into the part of the patient's body that needs healing or improvement. Growth factors contained in this portion of the blood stimulate the stem cells in the patient's body to mature into new and healthy adult cells that replace the damaged or diseased cells. This allows the tissues to heal.

A healthy individual, of course, heals faster than an unhealthy individual. Children heal faster than elderly people. To use the natural healing ability of the body to heal parts that are not as healthy as they could be is an exciting prospect, and is accessible since we all have these materials present in our bodies. It's something that is readily available and we don't need to manufacture it or buy it from somewhere else.

PRP has been used to heal different conditions:

- In cardiac surgery, PRP is used to heal an ailing heart.
- PRP can heal bone fractures.
- PRP has also been used to accelerate the healing of wounds.

PRP can also be applied to heal erectile tissue. Though its use in the treatment of ED is novel, PRP has been used for rejuvenation of tissues for some time. It can be used to rejuvenate any tissue or any part of the body that is not as healthy as it could be.

Growth Factors From the Patient's Blood

Human blood consists of different parts:

- Red and white blood cells
- Particles called *platelets*
- A liquid portion called *plasma*

The platelets, which are small particles in the blood, contain different types of growth factors. The white blood cells, platelets, and the plasma are the parts of the blood used for the PRP.

The red blood cells carry oxygen around the body. But we don't use that portion of the blood for the PRP.

This means that the red blood cells have to be separated from the plasma, the platelets, and the white blood cells, which is done by spinning the blood in a centrifuge.

Usually, it is also necessary to activate the growth factor in the platelets by adding a salt solution — *calcium chloride* — that is normally found in the body, and this causes the platelets to release the growth factors. When you have an injury, some substances, including calcium chloride, are released at the site of the injury. This activates the growth factors in the platelets to start healing the injured tissue by stimulating young immature cells to develop into new, healthy adult cells. This same principle applies when we are using PRP in a procedure to heal. The calcium chloride, or in some cases another salt solution known as *calcium gluconate*, is used to activate or release the growth factors from the platelets.

These growth factors then stimulate the stem cells. Stem cells are found in every tissue: they are dormant, immature cells. The growth factors stimulate these stem cells to start maturation and grow into new and healthy adult cells. These adult cells will then replace the damaged or diseased cells in that area. This will apply to any tissue in the body.

Effect of the Growth Factor on Immature Cells in Penile Tissue

The growth factors that have been released from the platelets by adding the salt or activator will stimulate the stem cells in the penile tissue. The penile tissue has blood vessels, fibroblasts, elastic tissues, and stem cells. By injecting the growth factors into the penile tissue, the stem cells mature into adult cells lining the inside of the blood vessel, and the fibroblasts are activated and stimulated to mature into adult cells. These adult cells will then replace the damaged mature cells that cause ED in the erectile tissue. The damage caused by high blood pressure or diabetes or other small-vessel diseases can be reversed, by stimulating new and healthier mature cells to develop the blood vessels and other tissues.

The same healing properties will apply to stem cells in patients who have had nerve injuries. By using the growth factors in the cell and stimulating the development of these young cells, the penile tissue can be rejuvenated to a level where the function could be much better than it was before.

Stem cells can also heal scarring in the penile tissue, which sometimes develops after the removal of an implant or from some other cause, like Peyronie's disease. The growth factors, by activating the stem cells and leading to the development of new healthier adult cells, can help heal the tissue in these other conditions.

THE P-SHOT: DESCRIBED

One of the advantages of the Priapus Shot or P-Shot is that it is a minimally invasive procedure. Before we do any procedure at BodyLogicMD of Houston, we make sure that you understand the process and have the opportunity to ask questions. After the consultation, an informed consent is obtained based on the information we have provided. You are then taken into a comfortable procedure room and lie on the couch.

The area for the blood draw is cleansed, and the method will be similar to a regular blood draw; the difference is that since the blood is going to be reinjected into the patient, the procedure has to be sterile and the blood needs to be collected in a sterile tube. In a regular blood draw, the area is wiped with an alcohol wipe, and then the blood is drawn, while in this case, we actually use a much stronger cleansing solution to clean the site of the blood draw.

Usually, blood is drawn from the veins in the front of the elbow, unless the veins there are difficult to access. In such a case, blood will be drawn from any other readily accessible vein. Sometimes, local anesthesia is applied to the area of the blood draw to make the entire procedure as painless as possible. The blood is drawn into a tube that contains anticoagulants to prevent the blood from clotting.

The drawn blood is put into a special tube and spun in a centrifuge. The spinning separates the red blood cells, which are heavier, to settle in the bottom of the tube, and then the plasma and the platelets (containing the growth factors) and the white blood cells can be accessed from the top of the tube.

Anesthesia cream is applied to the penis before the blood draw takes place. Sometimes the sensory nerve to the penis can be blocked with local anesthetic injection. This gives the anesthesia enough time to act, up to ten minutes, and get the area numb. The numbing from the anesthesia will usually last for only two hours.

After the blood has been spun, the PRP, the straw-colored top layer of the spun blood, is separated from the red blood cells. This is the portion used for the procedure.

That portion is then divided into three parts. Usually the procedure will use at least 8–10 mL of this PRP for a single P-Shot. The PRP is now divided into portions for injecting into different areas of the penis during the procedure.

At this stage, the platelets have not been activated to release the growth factor. This is done just a few seconds before the injection because, if it is done too soon, the PRP will clot. When clotting occurs, it becomes very difficult to complete the procedure without having to use a large bore needle, which would be simply unacceptable.

The PRP is divided into two amounts:

- 1 mL is obtained to be injected into the glans penis.

- 2 mL will be injected at two points along the shaft of the penis, close to the base and toward the glans on either side.

Remember, we have applied topical anesthesia, so this is quite painless.

The penis and the surrounding area are of course cleansed thoroughly with antiseptic solution to sterilize the area before the injection. After the area has been cleaned and the drape placed to isolate it from the surrounding parts of the body, 2 mL of the PRP is then activated with about 0.2–0.3 mL of the activating agent, which in this case is calcium chloride.

The 2mL portion of activated PRP is injected into the end of the shaft towards the base of the penis. The injections are at the sides at three o'clock and nine o'clock positions.

The 1 mL that has been dedicated for the glans injection is now activated and injected across the glans, close to the junction with the shaft on the tip of the penis toward the junction to the shaft.

Some patients may feel a little pressure during the injections. We inject the solution as slowly as possible, without allowing the PRP to clot, to avoid a sudden increase in pressure and unnecessary discomfort.

If any injection site bleeds, which is uncommon, the bleeding is stopped by applying pressure. At this stage, the PRP procedure has been completed.

We like to have the patient use a penile pump immediately afterward; the pump is an FDA-approved penile pump used for ED. The pump is set at a specific negative pressure, which in this case is 10 mmHg—millimeters of mercury, a measurement of pressure—and is applied for ten minutes.

Why do we do this?

First, the negative pressure helps spread the PRP injection evenly throughout the penile tissue. Second, the negative pressure acts like a mild injury to the penis. Since the body's natural reaction is to try to heal an injury, that semblance of mild injury then attracts the healing factors in the blood to the area, and the stem cells are even more activated to try to heal this trauma. This way, the effect of the PRP is enhanced or increased.

The patient is then advised to use the pump twice a day, ten minutes each time, at ten mmHg of pressure for at least four weeks. After that, for the next two to four weeks, the pump is used once a day.

This is the PRP procedure in brief.

What do we hope to achieve with this?

1. The stem cells from the blood vessels will be activated.

2. The stem cells from the connective tissue fibroblasts will be activated.

3. Neural or nerve stem cells will also be activated.

All this put together will help to heal the erectile tissue.

After the procedure it is recommended that patients use some nutritional supplements that can increase blood flow in the small blood vessels and therefore enhance the blood supply to the penile tissue. Some doctors might recommend that patients use ED medications for a few days: ten days to two weeks after the procedure.

I prefer that my patients use natural products that are going to do the same thing without side effects.

Also, in preparation for the PRP, my patients sometimes are required to use supplements to improve their growth factors, as this will also improve their results.

EXPECTATIONS AND RESULTS

No matter what medical procedure is undertaken, it is important for a patient to be informed and to have realistic expectations. You can only have realistic expectations if the practitioner is careful not to exaggerate the possibility of positive results. When patients know what to expect, that gives them a good opportunity to decide if they are willing to do the procedure and hope for the best, but also willing to accept whatever results they get. In most procedures, it is very important to manage expectations.

Individual Results Vary

Individual results vary depending on a patient's age. Younger patients will have healthier stem cells, so the results usually are better in younger patients. When I say *younger patients*, I mean a forty-something-year-old man, who could expect to have healthier stem cells than an eighty-something-year-old man.

Of course, calendar years are not the only factor to consider when evaluating the age of a person's tissues. When I say forty years old, I am referring to a forty-year-old who has lived a healthy life and does not have any serious health conditions.

The other important factor is the original cause of ED. A person who is unable to control his diabetes or is a chain smoker who has had a great deal of tissue damage or blood vessel damage could not expect to have the same results as a young person who has had problems that are either minimal or well controlled.

However, if the ED is the result of major trauma, then the results may not be as good as for someone who has not experienced tissue damage in the area.

This is not to say that these people will not experience some positive results. They simply may need multiple procedures to achieve significant results. For example, a patient who has had complications from prostate surgery may fall into a group that will need multiple procedures to experience a positive outcome.

At BodyLogicMD of Houston, we have had experience with a patient who had prostate surgery and then improved his erectile function by 60 percent after just one Priapus Shot treatment, because this patient was quite healthy otherwise.

The results you expect will depend upon how healthy the individual is, because the healthier you are, the healthier your stem cells are, the healthier your platelets are, and the more effective the growth factors will be. Furthermore, the less damaged the tissues are, the more easily they can be repaired.

Improvement After Initial Treatment: 20–60 Percent Positive Results

Based on the general health of the patient and the patient's ability to heal, most men can expect to experience about 20–60 percent improvement in erectile function after the initial Priapus Shot. The healthier an individual is, the less likely it is that their ED is due to major small blood vessel damage. But if the severity of their problem is due to injury or surgery, then they may not achieve 60 percent improvement and may have results in between 20 and 60 percent. There are always individual variations in the results.

A healthy person will always heal better and faster. For any kind of surgery, if one patient is anemic and another isn't, the person who is not anemic is going to come out of the surgery much better than the person with anemia. When you come to me to have a P-Shot done, I stress the fact that your results will be as good as your lifestyle or any changes that you are willing and able to make and maintain. I always encourage my patients to be conscious and maintain their health.

Initial Improvement Can Be a Volume Effect

A patient usually will notice some changes in either their erectile function or in the size of the penis. A lot of that initial improvement is transient and due to the 9–10 mL of PRP that has been injected into the area. As the fluid gets absorbed into the blood vessels and goes into other parts of the body, that effect will diminish.

When the patient knows what is going on, then they do not become unnecessarily worried about a poor result. The increase in volume may disappear or be reduced, but the platelets and growth factors have yet to do their jobs: to stimulate the patient's stem cells. The patient should expect this initial improvement to diminish over a few days to a week.

Actual Effect of PRP Begins Four Weeks After the Procedure

The actual effect of PRP is seen when the growth factors stimulate the stem cells to start developing into new, mature adult cells. This does not start until about three to four weeks after the procedure. That is when stem cells start to mature, and it may take as long as three months for the stem cells to fully mature into their adult form.

Usually, you will be advised that the actual effect of the PRP starts at about four weeks and will continue until about three months. That may extend until six months. The effect at six months is the maximum effect that you can expect to receive from that procedure.

Fortunately, you retain what improvements you have already gained from the procedure, so long as you do not continue the lifestyle or habits that caused the ED and made the procedure necessary in the first place: chain smoking, or not doing anything to control diabetes, or not making any effort to protect yourself when you are involved in contact sports.

If the patient needs an augmentation of the Priapus Shot, this can be done after three months, but preferably between three and six months after the initial procedure. This will then augment or add on to the results from the previous procedure.

Final Results

By six months, most of the stem cells in the penile tissue that have been activated by the Priapus Shot will have developed into their mature adult forms. Any stem cells that haven't been stimulated by the PRP will probably not be stimulated without another injection of the PRP or growth factors.

If you would like to improve your results, then six months after the intial procedure would be the optimal time to do the second procedure.

But I stress to my clients that while repeating the PRP could improve the results, I still think that your tissues or anyone's tissues are as healthy as you allow them to be. Anything that you or any of us can do to keep ourselves healthy can improve the results of PRP or any surgical procedure.

It is important to manage your expectations, and the best way to improve your expectations is to stay healthy in all ways. Sometimes, we prepare our patients by giving them supplements that improve the production of their growth factors. Others who have chronic diseases such as diabetes and high blood pressure are also counseled on what they could do to improve control of these diseases. Of course, the smokers need to stop smoking. Remember, ED informs the patient about the patient about what is happening to other blood vessels in the body, including the brain and the heart.

To improve the blood supply to the penis after the procedure, everything and anything that you can do to keep the blood vessels and other parts of your body healthy is highly recommended. This will include:

- Limiting fast foods and empty calories
- Eating nutritious food

- Supplements with micronutrients: vitamins and minerals

All of the nutrients we need for a healthy body and complete healing can be found in the foods we eat. If we eat healthy, whole foods we will need fewer items from the supplement shop.

We know that nicotine is highly addictive and that smokers have difficulties in changing this habit, but it is of utmost importance that they do so. It is advised that a smoker seek help to achieve this.

For men who are chronically stressed, especially younger patients, their ED is most likely stress-related. These patients should speak to somebody who could help them manage their chronic stress. Or they can do something themselves. They can meditate, pray, get massages, take walks, and learn tai chi, yoga, or qi gong. Even having a salt bath can help a person to de-stress. Counsel yourself positively. All the above will improve results and ensure that you maintain the results that you have achieved.

Other Uses of the P-Shot

The P-Shot can be used to treat other conditions involving the penis, for example, to heal scar tissues caused by *Peyronie's disease*. This is a condition that affects the penile shaft with scaring. This is associated with abnormal curvatures and deformities during erection. The actual cause is unknown. Injuries, surgery, advancing age, or genetics have been implicated.

Scarring can also be caused by injury to the penis or surgery to remove penile implants. It is also used to achieve penile enlargement. For these patients, the use of a penile pump is mandatory, and repeat procedures are usually necessary to achieve the maximum result.

CHAPTER *FOUR*

Can I Improve My Results?

FACTORS AFFECTING OUTCOMES

There are a number of actions you can take to affect the degree of improvement that you obtain from the Priapus Shot. Some of the following actions are to be taken by you, and others are for your healthcare practitioner.

Root Causes

The cause of ED can affect the results you obtain from treatment. For example, if the ED is caused by an ongoing health issue, then the best results would be obtained if that health issue is either removed or its effect is reduced. If, on the other hand, the ED is caused by severe trauma, then because of the extent of the injury, it might take more effort to get the result both the practitioner and the patient are expecting. All of these issues will need to be explained, addressed, and understood before the procedure so the expectations for the results are realistic.

Lifestyle Habits

Lifestyle habits can be toxic to the human body:

- Smoking
- Recreational drug use
- Alcohol use
- Poor diet

Bad lifestyle choices can also lead to chronic diseases:

- Diabetes
- High blood pressure
- Autoimmune diseases

These would compound the small blood vessel issues as well as problems in other cells functioning in the body.

LIFESTYLE FACTORS

It's important to discuss lifestyle factors because there are things you can do as an individual to improve your overall health and therefore the result of any procedure that is done.

Many patients think that their doctor is responsible for their health. That's not the case. Your doctor can act as a coach to guide you through your journey to good health, but it is up to you, the individual, to do what you can to maintain your health. For example, your doctor may recommend that you change what you eat, or advise you to eat something specific. It is your choice, your responsibility, to follow the advice; the doctor will not eat the food for you.

So if you want to attain the benefits of eating healthful foods, sleeping well, avoiding toxic substances like alcohol and tobacco, and practicing meditation, you have to actually do these things. Your healthcare provider cannot do them for you.

Smoking

I mentioned earlier in this chapter that smoking is one of the most toxic things you can do to yourself. The abuse to the cells in the body comes from:

- The smoke itself, or the hydrocarbons that are produced by burning tobacco

- Nicotine, a dangerously addictive substance

- Heavy metal poisoning (from arsenic, lead, cadmium) in the additives of manufactured cigarettes

The nicotine causes blood vessels to constrict. The constriction of these blood vessels has the greatest affect on the smallest blood vessels.

If a chronic or chain-smoker has ED issues, then the continuous poisoning of his blood vessels must be addressed. To get any significant benefits from such a treatment, you must remove that additional risk. Stopping smoking, or at least making an effort to reduce the number of cigarettes, would help improve the results of a PRP procedure for this patient.

All these toxic assaults from cigarettes cause damage to your body's cells and cause inflammation. The inflammation can have other far-reaching effects on your health. The effects of the cigarette smoke can cause cells to start behaving abnormally and become cancerous.

Smoking is a terrible habit. I accept that it is a habit that is difficult to break. However, every attempt should be made to break that habit since it affects everything in a patient's life, even the results of the P-Shot procedure.

For patients who smoke, please be aware that it is usually more difficult to obtain the blood that is needed for the procedure. In a nonsmoker, it may take as little as five seconds to get into the vein and draw the blood. It may take twenty to thirty minutes to find a vein in a smoker. If the outside veins are that difficult to find, you could imagine what is happening to the smaller blood vessels.

Bad Food Choices

Bad food choices are toxic to the body. Poor diet can also lower your testosterone level.

If you eat a lot of processed food, it actually causes the body to lose essential nutrients in order to digest and deal with these inadequate foods:

- Donuts, pancakes, pretzels, breakfast biscuits with refined flours and sugars

- Processed foods high in sodium

- Cold-cut meats with nitrates and nitrites added for preservation

When it comes to diet, the intake of processed foods or processed meats increases inflammation and free radical damage in the body. That affects the small blood vessels everywhere in the body, including in the penile tissue. To improve your results after the PRP procedure, you can address these issues in your diet. Improve what you eat so that you don't continue exacerbating the original problem that the PRP procedure is supposed to have treated.

The net result of eating fast foods is therefore a deficit. It is like being handed a counterfeit note and giving back genuine currency in return. All this does in the body is allow an excessive amount of sugar to float around. While the pancreas is still able, it will make enough insulin to take care of the excess blood sugar. However, some of this blood sugar will attach to proteins, and these could be proteins from any part of the body. The attachment of this sugar to tissues disrupts the functioning of the tissues and increases silent inflammation, a slow rusting effect that, if not controlled, will damage tissues.

Inflammation can make the blood vessels stiffer and unable to dilate normally. The inflammation can also destroy the inner lining of the blood vessels, compromising the blood supply to the area. Eventually, this individual will become diabetic. For more about the important role of insulin, healthy blood sugar levels, and diabetes, see the following section, "Hormone Imbalance and Chronic Disease."

On the flip side, when you eat a balanced diet, with enough complex carbohydrates, adequate protein, and adequate healthy fats, you will nurture your body and reduce inflammation and reduce the chances of developing diabetes and other complications.

Sports

Being physically active is well known to be good for your body, but sports, even noncontact sports, can also pose the risk of injury. For example, a baseball player should wear protective coverings, including in the pelvic area. A fastball can cause a lot of damage to the groin.

A cyclist puts a lot of pressure on the internal pudendal artery and the perineal vein as well as other vessels and nerves in the pelvic area. A good-quality seat can reduce the chances of severe injury in the pelvic area, which may also involve the penis and the erectile tissue.

Wearing adequate protective gear and not indulging in dangerous sports activities can reduce the chances of an injury in the first place. Prevention is always better than a cure, so we should do all we can to prevent injury to any part of the body, including the penile tissues.

Substance Abuse and Illicit Drug Use

A lot of illicit drugs cause constriction of blood vessels in many parts of the body.

These drugs include:

- Cocaine
- Methamphetamine
- Crack

In time, the effects on blood vessels can undermine any positive results that might be experienced from the Priapus treatment. For an individual who uses any of these types of drugs, they should also expect to have some problems down the road. Yes, they can have a P-Shot, but they are not likely to get the same results as somebody whose blood vessels are healthier than theirs.

Removing the predisposing cause is always important to improve the results from this procedure.

Why try to put out a fire while another person pours gasoline on it?

This is what is happening if these individuals do not change their lifestyle habits.

Recreational drug use can also affect outcomes, with symptoms such as:

- Constriction of the blood vessels
- Effects on hormone production
- Increased inflammation

Excessive alcohol use will affect the body because of increased inflammation and hormone suppression. This will also compound the problem with the small blood vessels. Cutting back on alcohol intake will most likely increase a patient's chance of getting a good result from the PRP procedure.

Stress and Lack of Sleep

Chronic stress can be caused by many things, including a lack of sleep. But chronic stress can also be mental, emotional, or physical.

Chronic stress affects how the body works and the body's production of essential hormones, including testosterone, which is very important in erectile function. In addition, chronic stress increases cortisol production. An excess of cortisol, even though this is a hormone that sustains life, will cause tissue damage. For more about the importance of balanced cortisol, see the following section, "Hormone Balance."

The ultimate effects of chronic stress on the body include:

- Disruption of most ordinary functions, including hormone production

- Increased inflammation

- Decreased ability to recover from any type of injury

- In the case of younger patients, low testosterone

- Anxiety

Anxiety associated with chronic stress can also prevent a young man from achieving an erection. It is extremely important to address stress. If a particular stress can be avoided, it should be.

Certain stresses cannot be avoided. If the stress is related to a job, and you are not in a position to change your job immediately, then there is not much you can do. If you leave your job, you will only experience even more stress.

So the best approach is to manage the stress. Two individuals can be given the same source of stress and react in completely different ways. It is possible to train yourself to react to the difficulties in life in more effective ways; meditation, prayer, yoga, or massage may be helpful. Some men may feel that an inward, body-centered practice such as yoga is not masculine, but they may be surprised to learn that in India, where yoga comes from, men have traditionally studied and taught yoga for centuries.

Chronic stress can cause cancer by destroying the body's ability to defend itself or to function properly, so I reiterate: it is important to address chronic stress.

There are three very important factors that you can control to reduce the chances of developing ED or chronic diseases:

1. Adopt healthy lifestyle practices, such as following a nutritionally sound diet.

2. Avoid destructive habits to maintain health and prevent disease.

3. Develop strategies for dealing with chronic stress.

If doing this on your own proves difficult, we can help you. See the "Next Steps" section for how to contact us. Successfully making changes in the factors listed above increases the likelihood of better results from a treatment like the P-Shot.

We have a saying in functional medicine:

Lifestyle trumps any medication or treatment that a patient could be given.

In the case of diabetes, for example, it does not matter how many pills the patient takes; if he does not also change his lifestyle and reduce the load of excessive sugar and carbohydrate intake on the body, he will not achieve optimal health. Diabetics who can work on their lifestyle tend to need less medication as time goes by. A patient should do whatever he himself can do to reduce the need for procedures and extra medications.

We are bombarded with messages on various media, to "ask your doctor if this is right for you" whenever a new medication is approved by the FDA.

But patients also need to hear the message, "This is what you can do for yourself so that you *don't* need to ask your doctor if a certain medication is right for you."

HORMONE IMBALANCE AND CHRONIC DISEASE

Several hormones will affect the small blood vessels in the body, especially sex hormones. Sex hormones affect the health of the small blood vessels. When I say sex hormones, I mean *testosterone* for men and *estrogen* for women. However, in men, the conversion of testosterone into estrogen in the cell lining of the small blood vessels is important.

If a man is deficient in testosterone and cannot maintain the usual activity of protecting the function of his testosterone in the small blood vessels of any part of the body, including the penile tissue, the heart, or the brain, then he is not going to get the expected results from the PRP procedures. For a man to spend money for the PRP procedure while his hormones are depleted would be shortchanging himself, because the result would be less than he could have experienced if his levels were normal.

Also, if a man is low in testosterone and is using ED medication, the results can be less satisfactory.

Insulin

As mentioned earlier in this chapter, another hormone that affects the small blood vessels in the body is insulin. For diabetics whose tissues have lost sensitivity to insulin or who are unable to make enough insulin, the continuously high levels of glucose in their blood will damage cells and cause inflammation. This will affect the cells lining the small blood vessels everywhere in the body.

To be able to experience a proper result from the PRP procedure, the diabetes needs to be better controlled.

Steps you can take for effective treatment of diabetes include:

- Follow your healthcare provider's orders.
- Take the prescribed medications.
- Be cautious about the foods in your diet.
- Exercise regularly.

By improving your control over diabetes, you are reducing the chances of complications like small blood vessel problems or diseases, and then you will improve the results you are likely to get from the PRP procedure. You can also ensure that any new tissues will not be damaged by high blood sugar.

Since testosterone is involved in our ability to metabolize glucose and carbohydrates, men should look at testosterone as something to help with blood sugar control. Diabetes is more common in men with low testosterone.

Cortisol

Cortisol is another very important hormone that you need to survive, but too much of it is not healthy and too little is just as bad. Cortisol is important for energy generation during fight-or-flight situations. It is important for your immune system and proper functioning of other hormones in the proper amount. Excess cortisol will increase weight gain and suppress the immune system.

Hormones are very important for the proper functioning of the human body. Every function in your body needs balance to maintain health.

Getting It Just Right

Too much of a good thing is not necessarily good. Too little of a good thing is not good either. The body works best when following a Goldilocks-like pattern: not too much, not too little, the amount needs to be *just right*.

Properly balanced hormones improve the body's ability to heal and protect itself from ongoing stresses and toxins. For example, if, as a diabetic, you do not change your lifestyle, the conventional treatment plan is to take insulin. However, the insulin itself is also toxic to the body. Yes, you need insulin to deal with high rates of blood sugar, but you need only just enough insulin. Extra insulin might cause more problems.

In men, testosterone maintains the health of blood vessels through its conversion into estrogen. Excessive estrogen can result in unhealthy blood vessels. Deficient testosterone can result in diseased or unhealthy blood vessels.

Low testosterone results in the inability of the man to maintain the health of the *endothelium* — the interior lining of blood vessels — to serve as an interface between the blood and the surrounding blood vessel wall. Low testosterone will result in abnormal or inadequate functioning of these cells, which will then affect the ability of the blood vessels to dilate.

However, not everyone with low testosterone needs to have a hormone supplement. It is important to discover precisely why a man's testosterone is low and address that factor first of all.

When the other factors associated with the activity of the testosterone have not been addressed, testosterone can produce other hormones in the body like estrogen and *dihydotestosterone*, DHT. As stated before, these need to be in the right balance and therefore should be evaluated regularly.

Especially if you are a young man, there are many steps you can take to improve hormonal health:

- Exercise using resistance training.
- Clean up your diet.
- Practice stress relief.
- Avoid and remove toxins (from smoking, food, or environment)

It is important that young men have their hormones in balance.

Hormone Replacement and Supplementation

For some men, lifestyle changes can improve the production of testosterone. Others, especially older men, may need to supplement their testosterone. With age, the ability to make testosterone diminishes. There is a lot of confusing information about the safety of hormone replacement therapy.

If your chosen route of treatment is hormone replacement or supplementation, you must have the guidance of a practitioner who knows how to do this safely and properly. If the testosterone dosage is too high, for instance, it will very likely to lead to more production of estrogen. If your provider writes you a prescription for testosterone supplementation for a year, but doesn't monitor your levels by checking them at least twice in that year, they have not done you any favors.

You cannot be injected with testosterone without follow-up and expect to receive the full benefit; there are side effects if the supplementation is not done properly. If you are on testosterone supplementation, regular monitoring will ensure you are getting the maximum benefit of the treatment and none of the side effects. Do not opt out of visiting your healthcare provider to save a few dollars at the cost of your health.

I am a firm believer that hormones do not cause cancer on their own, but that the way your body handles hormones, either naturally produced or prescribed hormones, can lead to cancer. So be sure to receive your hormone supplementation from someone who knows how to evaluate these factors and correct them if necessary.

The other hormone involved in erectile function is DHT. Under certain situations, the patient may not make enough of this. This could be improved with a change to healthier dietary habits.

There are some supplements that could improve the balance between the estrogen and the dihydrotestosterone. We never like a man to have too much estrogen, but he has to have enough because that is needed for brain function, too. Men need the female hormone estrogen to think. However it has to be just enough, not too much.

In addition to playing a primary role in sexual activity and maintaining erectile function, testosterone:

- Controls blood sugar
- Builds muscles
- Builds bones
- Regulates the immune system
- Controls pain and helps raise pain tolerance

Supporting and Sustaining the Effects of the P-Shot

After the procedure, there are nutritional supplements that can help improve the health of small blood vessels. It may be necessary for you to take these, at least in the period following the procedure, to augment any benefits that you receive from the actual PRP P-Shot procedure.

These would be the types of supplements that:

- Reduce inflammation
- Increase nitric oxide production
- Improve blood flow to an area, which can heal the damage of blood vessels either through nitric oxide production or simply by relaxing the muscles in the larger blood vessels that lead to the small ones

Even something as simple as a good-quality omega-3 fish oil would help to improve the results of the P-Shot.

There are lots of other good nutritional supplements that could help improve the health of the small blood vessels, and I recommend them for my patients:

- Alpha Lipoic Acid
- Co-Q10
- Nitrogenesis
- Neogenesis
- Amino Acids, like Citrulin
- Magnesium Glycinate/Taurate
- Supplements that aid blood sugar management
- Berberin
- Chromium Polynicoyinate
- Vitamin D3
- Supplements that can support testosterone production, like Tonghat Ali

It may also be necessary to use some erectile function enhancing supplements, or it may be necessary for you to take ED medication just to make sure that you are getting increased blood supply to the area.

CHAPTER *FIVE*

Who Can Benefit From Erectile Dysfunction Treatment?

EFFECTS ON THE PATIENT

The effects of diseases and health problems in general most often do not affect only the individual suffering from the disease or health problem. Your health has an impact on the people around you. In order to minimize the negative emotional impact on the people around you, it is important to realize that these effects exist and address them. This may also help the individuals around you to be more understanding and empathetic toward you, in return.

It can also help you to be more aware of how your health problems affect others. You can then make a conscious effort to limit the negative impact on the people around you, realizing that they are not responsible for your problems. Making other people unhappy because you are overwhelmed with the problem does not deal with the problem. It just makes everyone around you miserable.

Emotional Toll Can Lead to Other Diseases

Patients with erectile dysfunction are usually under some stress. ED itself could be the result of chronic stress. This could be compounded by worry or anxiety regarding the inability to perform. There is performance-associated stress from the real problem, ED, compounded by the additional stress of the anticipated problem.

We know that stress is a great killer. Chronic stress can lead to all sorts of health problems, including chronic diseases like diabetes. In situations of chronic stress the body does not react as well as it should. We know that chronic stress can lead to cancer, autoimmune diseases, and depression, and other emotional issues, and it can also lead to dementia. We usually recommend that patients do whatever is necessary to eliminate chronic stress. When one cannot eliminate the chronic stress, one should at least do something to minimize the effect of chronic stress on the body.

ED in this situation can be treated or at least addressed and managed with different options, as mentioned in an earlier chapter of the book. It is important for the patient to realize that there is no need for him to be chronically stressed when there is help available.

Lack of Self-Confidence

A man with ED not only lacks self-confidence when he is around his significant other, but also when he is around his male friends. He could still be a fairly confident man but compared to his former self, his self-esteem could have dropped quite a bit. Somehow, at the back of the patient's mind he may wonder if his problem is obvious to others. Even if he doesn't imagine that others suspect that he has a problem, he may think that everyone around him is performing better than they actually are, which is another figment of his imagination, because the man he is next to may possibly have a much more serious issue.

A man who suffers from ED may become reluctant to join in activities that he would have enjoyed before. Again, because ED is a treatable and manageable condition, nobody should have to go through social isolation and embarrassment. Help is at hand.

Poor Drive, Poor Outlook, and Inferior Job Performance

A patient with poor confidence, a patient who is chronically stressed, or a patient who is depressed will have low initiative and ambition. When a person has poor drive, their job performance suffers. The confident man who has a problem can at least do something about this problem. But when a patient does not have self-confidence, the fear of failure makes them unwilling to try. And sometimes the fear of failure will cause the individual to not make an attempt to try to do the job or project at hand. This leads to underproduction, both for the individual and for whatever group he is working for.

If you are an entrepreneur, this can be an even more serious problem, because when you work for yourself, you eat what you kill, so to speak. If you are unable to perform, then you are not killing much, and you won't be eating much, either. On the other hand, this affects all of the people around you, especially if you have a family to support.

The other effect of ED on the patient is anxiety. You may become an anxious, chronically stressed man, with a chip on your shoulder. You may become more angry and tend to overreact and blow up, and that's not only unhealthy for you, but it could also be unsafe for the people around you. Since this is a treatable problem, even if the result is not 100 percent improvement, there are options for you to try. A P-Shot is one of the best and least invasive procedures that could be offered to a patient who qualifies for the treatment.

EFFECTS ON SPOUSE AND FAMILY

There is a spiritual and electrical connection between individuals, and we all have an electrical or force field surrounding each of us. Our mood affects everyone who gets within that field. If you are around a happy person, then you tend to be happier than if you are around a depressed or anxious or irritable person. Everybody in the field of someone with any of the emotional factors discussed earlier is bound to have these negative emotions rub off on them.

The spouse and the children of the patient with ED and any associated emotional issues may try to avoid him because of the alarming changes that they sense in him. The man who is distressed over his ED and health problems may be unpleasant and difficult to please. He will be no fun to be around. This carries over into the workplace. It is important to realize that the effect of ED is not limited to the individual. The emotional impact affects others around him.

Emotional Effect

The brunt of the emotional effect is on the spouse or significant other of this individual because they worry about the effect of ED on the man. There is also the issue of not gaining satisfaction from sexual activity. The case with most of the patients I've seen is that most of their worry is over their inability to satisfy their partners. This compounds the emotional stress caused by this problem, which fortunately is treatable. This causes unnecessary suffering for everyone: the patient and those around him.

Effect on Intimacy

The man with ED does not want to have intimate relations with their significant other because of the fear of failure. This becomes a major issue, not only for him, but also for the significant other or spouse.

We know that healthy, safe sex is important for a full, healthy, and enjoyable life. If the individual with ED is afraid to even try because he could fail, he's suffering physically and emotionally, and his intimate partner also suffers both emotionally and physically. Two individuals are now suffering because of this problem in one person. Again, that is unnecessary because there are options available for treating this problem. Even if the results are not always 100 percent improvement, they can still be very significant.

Involvement With Children

A stressed, irritable, angry man or one who has no self-confidence becomes like a chained animal. The children who are used to playing with their father, having fun with him and having discussions with him are now unable to do so because Dad is not willing to play. Dad is not in the mood to engage in family discussions because at the back of his mind, he has this overwhelming worry that he is no longer a man.

Fortunately, women do not have this severe emotional response to sexual dysfunction. Women do not have ED. Even if they have a lack of sex drive, they are typically not as devastated about it as the men are. For some reason, that's a man's second brain. When a man is unhappy, they don't interact well with people around him. Children are very perceptive. They will realize that Dad is not in the mood to play, but the children, especially if they are very young, won't understand why. They will start to wonder if they did something wrong. This is an issue that needs to be corrected for the sake of the mental health of every member of the family.

EFFECTS ON FRIENDS AND COWORKERS

It's important to stress the fact that the effect of ED on a person is not limited to only him and the people immediately around him. Most of a man's leisure time, if not spent with family, is with friends. A patient who is in a lousy mood or who is absent-minded because he is wondering whether his situation could get worse makes his friends work harder to engage in conversation and activities.

If you have a depressed, irritable friend, or a friend who has suddenly changed from the person you used to know, you worry. Worrying is a form of stress. Now the individual with ED has chronic stress associated with his ED and his friends have chronic stress from worrying about him.

Friends would prefer not to be in that situation. No one is looking for more stress when spending time with friends. It should be a relaxing and stress-relieving time together. When you are depressed, you may want to stay indoors. If you are irritable or critical, then the other people in your house may prefer that you leave, even if for a brief period.

Improving Relations in the Workplace

Most men spend most of their time, except time off, with coworkers. A man who is preoccupied with his own problems makes the workplace difficult for his coworkers, as well.

Also, when you are not in a great mood, your job performance probably suffers. Your colleagues may bear the brunt of your worries and fears over ED. If you are not pulling your weight in a group project, for example, the group does not do as well as they can and can only maintain progress if someone else is pitching in for you if you are underperforming.

If you are depressed, anxious, and irritable, it's likely that you're not the most delightful coworker. There's even more cause for concern if you are a manager, supervisor, foreman, or boss in charge of productivity, safety, and progress of a whole team.

If you're working with someone who is depressed, then it drains the air out of the room. That is not the most productive environment in any situation. The depressed individual also underperforms.

Also, individuals working around or for a man worrying about his ED with its emotional baggage may need his advice about a task but neglect to ask him because they are worried he will blow up. Jobs that could have been done properly before now have to be done over again because this individual is unapproachable. That is costly for everyone in the workplace in terms of time, money, and productivity.

Again, if you experience ED, it can have extensive ramifications on the people around you. My advice is to *do something about it*. You don't need to keep suffering and punishing the people around you, even if you are doing it unconsciously. The people around you definitely suffer from the effect that ED has on you.

Improve Engagement in Activities

ED can affect a person's enjoyment and engagement in other activities beyond sex.

A lot of men think that their ability to perform sexually is the ultimate test of their manhood. For such an individual, ED can be devastating. If they feel that this process that identifies them as men is no longer viable, then all the other activities that involve being a man, even sometimes participating in sports activities with the family or friends, may now feel like a chore.

A patient may think, *Should I be playing a man's game?*

Should I be doing a man's job?

Friends and coworkers may hesitate to approach the patient or invite him to partake in activities. This leaves this individual more isolated and even more depressed.

Fortunately, this is an issue that something can be done about. If it were a problem without treatment the story would be different. I recommend that men with ED at least do some research and find out what could be done or what type of help is accessible to them. There are plenty of options, of which the P-Shot is one of the best and one of the least invasive.

Though the scenarios described above may occur only in the most extreme cases—with younger individuals and more emotionally fragile persons — it is still very important to address the mild to moderate cases of ED so that they do not become more severe.

Make some lifestyle changes that will stop the situation from getting worse.

Conclusion

In conclusion, I would like to stress again the fact that ED is a very common health problem. it can be caused by several factors. Many of the causes can be either prevented or treated.

It is also important that, because of the different options available for treating ED, there be an informed decision regarding what approach to take. I strongly recommend the P-Shot, which uses the natural healing ability of the body to correct the problem in the erectile tissue that is a root cause of the ED.

Apart from making the correct choice of treatment, it is also important to understand that the problem of ED affects more than the individual who has the problem. Dealing with the issue not only benefits the individual with ED but also benefits the people around him, including close family members, friends, significant others, and coworkers.

This being the case, ED treatment should be seriously considered by the patient, especially with a procedure that is minimally invasive, such as the P-Shot. Also because of the preventable causes of ED, a strong effort should be made by every patient to prevent diseases. If the problem has already manifested, find out what can be done to reduce the impact of the disease so that the complications that arise from the chronic existence of these diseases do not affect the optimal functioning of different parts of the body.

Also, it is important for those individuals to understand that ED is usually associated with a lot of chronic diseases like diabetes, high blood pressure, or autoimmune diseases. It is just the tip of the iceberg as a lot of destructive problems could be going on below the surface in the individual's body. An individual with ED should also find out the cause, if possible. Looking seriously for the cause could help the healthcare provider to uncover some more serious chronic health problems that can be addressed, thus potentially saving the patient's life. I have this discussion during all my consultations with patients for the P-Shot. I actually ask the patients to bring in their most recent labs to their appointment.

Safe, healthy lifestyle choices can have a positive, lifelong impact on erectile function and on the blood vessels of other parts of the body. Smokers should take the fact that they have ED as an eye-opener that something serious is happening with the blood vessels in the rest of the body. That should be an incentive to make a serious effort to stop smoking. It is not easy to stop smoking, but at least understanding the serious impact of smoking on the body could encourage some patients to make a concerted effort to quit.

Unfortunately, some smokers know that smoking can cause lung disease, emphysema, and other chronic problems, but that does not bother them. However, for a man, ED could be the one condition that could get his attention and convince him to do something about the smoking.

Remember, it is no use trying to put out a fire by pouring gasoline on it at the same time. Even after the patient has had treatment for ED with the P-Shot, continuing with the same habits or the same lifestyle factor that caused the problem in the first place would not be very helpful. Such behaviors will compromise the results.

A strong effort should be made by the patient to change his habits. Of course, it may be necessary for the people around him — family members, close friends, and even coworkers — to give him the support he needs to make a needed lifestyle change. This would also improve the end result he would get from treatment.

My practice focuses on optimizing the body's natural ability to heal and regenerate itself through lifestyle changes. We focus on all the areas that need to be addressed to achieve an extended health span: detoxification, nutrition, exercise, hormone balance, stress reduction, and sleep optimization. This program is available to all my patients, especially those with ED. This helps prevent or reduce the health impact of created, chronic diseases like diabetes.

Though I offer hormone replacement therapy, not everyone with low hormones needs supplementation. Most of the younger patients will just need to understand the cause of their low hormone production and address it. Not everyone with "Low T" will need testosterone.

ED may also be the driving force that brings men to doctors, as we know most men don't like to see doctors.

As much as it would be good not to have ED, it could be a blessing in the long run because it makes it possible for a healthcare practitioner to pick up on any other ongoing, potentially life-threatening health problems.

The takeaway from this book is for you to realize that ED is very common. There is help available, but if you don't ask for help, you won't get any. Recall that there are different ways to address ED, and that *less* is always *more*. It's always better to treat or manage any condition with the least aggressive option with the least potential side effect and as close to the healing process in nature as possible.

This is where the P-Shot comes in. Your own growth factors are used to stimulate immature cells, stem cells, to encourage them to develop into new and healthier adult cells, to heal the unhealthy tissue, which in this case, is the erectile tissue. With the P-Shot, the body's natural ability is stimulated in a very natural way to heal itself. This is the best option for treating certain types of ED.

Only when this does not achieve the desired result after an adequate span of time should more aggressive treatment be offered. Most procedures can be associated with complications. So if a condition needs to be treated, it should be treated with the procedure with the least chances of complications.

It's also important that while choosing what procedure a patient wants to have done, he does the research and makes sure that the practitioner who is going to do the treatment knows all about the problem, causes, and procedure.

You need to realize that the problem is not just a failure of erectile tissue to respond to sexual stimulus. There also may be other overwhelming factors in the body that need to be addressed at the same time. You should be prepared to take control of the aspects of your health that need attention in order to get the best results possible from your Priapus Shot.

When ED is related to emotional issues, for example, for a depressed young man who is in a conflicted relationship, it is important to address these issues, too, because depression and chronic stress can also lead to other chronic diseases, including cancer. ED can be improved either through counseling or trying to reduce the effects of chronic stress on the body. The patient should also be made to understand that the unnecessary chronic stress could cause more problems down the road than are currently evident, in this case their erectile functions.

If you have ED, do something about it.

Next Steps

BodyLogicMD of Houston, Texas, offers integrative and functional treatments for women and men with individualized wellness programs.

Call our office at 281-501-3666 or go to our website, www.priapusshot.com. to locate a properly trained provider near you.

About the Author

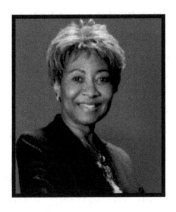

Dr. Okereke serves as Medical Director of BodyLogicMD of Houston, Texas, treating women and men with individualized wellness programs tailored to address each patient's specific, personal needs. Using a combination of integrative therapies, including customized nutrition and fitness regimens, pharmaceutical-grade supplementation, stress reduction techniques, and natural bioidentical hormone replacement therapy (BHRT), Dr. Okereke helps to restore her patients' energy levels, improve their mental clarity, and help them improve their overall health and health span.

Dr. Okereke transitioned into integrative and functional medicine to treat her patients using preemptive techniques to help them live the best life possible. Instead of using prescription drugs to treat a constellation of symptoms, Dr. Okereke helps her patients correct the underlying issues at their source. Dr. Okereke is a firm believer in the notion that the changes brought on by aging can be avoided or slowed with a well-balanced lifestyle.

Phyllis Okereke, MD, earned her medical degree from the University of Nigeria in 1975. After completing her internship, Dr. Okereke fulfilled her Residency in Ophthalmology in 1984. She is an active member of several professional medical organizations, including the Royal College of Ophthalmologists and the Royal College of Physicians and Surgeons. Dr. Okereke is also recognized as an active member of the American Academy of Anti-Aging and Regenerative Medicine, an active member of the Academy of Integrative Health and Medicine, and a Senior Fellow of the American Academy of Ophthalmology.

Dr. Okereke is a Diplomate of the American Board of Antiaging and Regenerative Medicine and the American Board of Integrative Holistic Medicine, and a member of the Academy of Integrative Health and Medicine. Dr. Okereke currently serves as Board Examiner for the American Board of Anti-Aging and Regenerative Medicine.

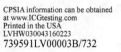

9 781945 446054